Second Edition

Workbook

Self-Care for New and Student Nurses

Dorrie K. Fontaine, PhD, RN, FAAN

Tim Cunningham, DrPH, MSN, RN, FAAN

Natalie May, PhD

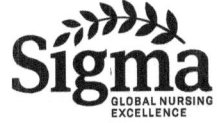

Copyright © 2025 by Sigma Theta Tau International Honor Society of Nursing

All rights reserved. This book is protected by copyright. No part of it may be reproduced, stored in a retrieval system, or transmitted in any form or by any means, electronic, mechanical, photocopying, recording, or otherwise, without written permission from the publisher. Any trademarks, service marks, design rights, or similar rights that are mentioned, used, or cited in this book are the property of their respective owners. Their use here does not imply that you may use them for a similar or any other purpose.

This book is not intended to be a substitute for the medical advice of a licensed medical professional. The author and publisher have made every effort to ensure the accuracy of the information contained within at the time of its publication and shall have no liability or responsibility to any person or entity regarding any loss or damage incurred, or alleged to have incurred, directly or indirectly, by the information contained in this book. The author and publisher make no warranties, express or implied, with respect to its content, and no warranties may be created or extended by sales representatives or written sales materials. The author and publisher have no responsibility for the consistency or accuracy of URLs and content of third-party websites referenced in this book.

Sigma Theta Tau International Honor Society of Nursing (Sigma) is a nonprofit organization whose mission is developing nurse leaders anywhere to improve healthcare everywhere. Founded in 1922, Sigma has more than 135,000 active members in over 100 countries and territories. Members include practicing nurses, instructors, researchers, policymakers, entrepreneurs, and others. Sigma's more than 540 chapters are located at more than 700 institutions of higher education throughout Armenia, Australia, Botswana, Brazil, Canada, Chile, Colombia, Croatia, England, Eswatini, Finland, Ghana, Hong Kong, Ireland, Israel, Italy, Jamaica, Japan, Jordan, Kenya, Lebanon, Malawi, Mexico, the Netherlands, Nigeria, Pakistan, Philippines, Portugal, Puerto Rico, Scotland, Singapore, South Africa, South Korea, Sweden, Taiwan, Tanzania, Thailand, the United States, and Wales. Learn more at www.sigmanursing.org.

Sigma Theta Tau International
550 West North Street
Indianapolis, IN, USA 46202

To request a review copy for course adoption, order additional books, buy in bulk, or purchase for corporate use, contact Sigma Marketplace at 888.654.4968 (US/Canada toll-free), +1.317.687.2256 (International), or solutions@sigmamarketplace.org.

To request author information, or for speaker or other media requests, contact Sigma Marketing at 888.634.7575 (US/Canada toll-free) or +1.317.634.8171 (International).

ISBN: 9781646482818
EPUB ISBN: 9781646482825
PDF ISBN: 9781646482832

Publisher: Dustin Sullivan
Acquisitions Editor: Emily Hatch
Development Editor: Jillmarie Leeper Sycamore
Cover Designer: Rebecca Batchelor
Interior Design/Page Layout: Rebecca Batchelor

Managing Editor: Carla Hall
Publications Specialist: Todd Lothery
Project Editor: Todd Lothery
Copy Editor: Erin Geile
Proofreader: Todd Lothery

About the Authors

Dorrie K. Fontaine, PhD, RN, FAAN, is the Dean Emerita at the University of Virginia (UVA) School of Nursing, where she served as Dean for 11 years until 2019. A champion of creating healthy work environments in clinical and academic settings, she is a past President of the American Association of Critical-Care Nurses (AACN). In 2009 she created the Compassionate Care Initiative at UVA, which has grown to be a guiding force in transforming the culture of the school with a focus on fostering human flourishing and resilience for students, faculty, and staff. A noted author of critical care texts, a leadership book, and multiple papers and presentations on creating healthy work environments through compassionate care, Fontaine credits a retreat at Upaya Zen Center in Santa Fe, New Mexico, with the Abbot, Roshi Joan Halifax, for setting her on the path of mindfulness, meditation, and a renewed focus on self-care. She attended Villanova University and the University of Maryland and received her PhD from The Catholic University of America. Her four-decade career of teaching and academic leadership includes the University of Maryland, Georgetown University, and the University of California, San Francisco. Working as a consultant with the Bedford Falls Foundation, she is now able to work with philanthropists who believe nurses are the future of healthcare. Fontaine lives in Charlottesville, Virginia, with her husband, Barry.

Tim Cunningham, DrPH, MSN, RN, FAAN, began his professional career as a performing artist and clown. He worked for two organizations that changed his life. The first, the Big Apple Circus, employed him to perform as a clown doctor at Boston Children's Hospital, Yale New Haven Children's Hospital, and Hasbro Children's Hospital. Concurrently, he volunteered for Clowns Without Borders (CWB), performing in various refugee camps, war zones, and other global zones of crisis. At the time of this publication, Tim is serving as Interim Executive Director of CWB. It was in pediatric hospitals and refugee camps where he witnessed and began to learn about the true meaning of resilience and self-care. The arts inspired him to pursue a career in nursing. He completed a second-degree nursing program at UVA and then became an emergency trauma nurse working clinically in Charlottesville, Virginia; Washington, DC; and New York City. It was during his time in New York that he completed his doctoral degree in public health at the Mailman School of Public Health at Columbia University. Cunningham is the former Director of the Compassionate Care Initiative at UVA, where he had the opportunity to work closely with Drs. Fontaine and May as the first edition of this book came to fruition. He currently lives in Atlanta, Georgia, where he established Emory Healthcare's Inaugural Office of Well-Being. While employed at Emory, he was Vice President, Co-Chief Well-Being Officer, and he also held a joint appointment as an Adjunct Associate Professor at the Nell Hodgson Woodruff School of Nursing at Emory University. Cunningham began his academic journey receiving his BA in English from the College of William and Mary in 2000. For self-care, Cunningham is an avid runner and wanna-be gardener. He loves any chance he can get to swim in the ocean or sit quietly as the sun rises.

Natalie May, PhD, transitioned to the UVA School of Nursing after 30 years as Associate Professor of Research in the Division of General Medicine in the UVA School of Medicine. She is a founding member of the UVA Center for Appreciative Practice. Certified as an Appreciative Inquiry facilitator and lead author of *Appreciative Inquiry in Healthcare,* she enjoys developing Appreciative Inquiry projects and teaching appreciative practice workshops at her home institution and beyond. She is an experienced qualitative researcher, and she has extensive experience in grant writing, program and curriculum development, and program evaluation. Her current research projects include the Mattering in Medicine study and the Mattering in Healthcare Education study. She was also an investigator for the Wisdom in Medicine Project: Mapping the Path Through Adversity to Wisdom, a study funded by the John Templeton Foundation. She is co-author of *Choosing Wisdom: The Path Through Adversity* and co-producer of a PBS film, *Choosing Wisdom*. She has co-developed and implemented an innovative curriculum for medical students, the Phronesis Project, designed to foster wisdom in young physicians, and she has implemented a similar program, Wisdom in Nursing, in the UVA School of Nursing. With Dorrie and Tim, she is lead author of *Self Care for Nurses: Small Doses for Wellness*. She earned a BA in economics and urban studies from Wellesley College, an MA in creative writing from Boston University, and her PhD in educational research from the UVA Curry School of Education. May lives in Richmond, Virginia, with her husband, Jim. Her most consistent and effective self-care practices are modern quilting and walking near water, especially the James River near her home and the ocean at the Outer Banks in North Carolina.

Contributing Authors

We would like to thank the following authors for their contributions to the book and their help in developing the exercises and prompts that form the essence of this workbook. We appreciate their diversity of experience and viewpoints.

Kim Acquaviva, PhD, MSW, CSE, FNAP (she/her)

Robin C. Brown-Haithco, MDiv (she/her)

Reynaldo "Ren" Capucao, Jr., MSN, RN, CNL (he/him)

Theresa Carroll, PhD (she/her)

Ebru Çayir, PhD, MD (she/her)

Roxana Chicas, PhD, RN (she/her)

Anna DeLong, MSW, LCSW, CEAP (she/her)

Susan Goins-Eplee, MSN, MDiv, RN, CNL, HEC-C (she/her)

Rosa Gonzalez-Guarda, PhD, MPH, RN, FAAN (she/her)

Julie Haizlip, MD, MAPP (she/her)

McKenzie Harper, MAT (she/her)

Susan Hassmiller, PhD, RN, FAAN (she/her)

Pamela Marie Hobby (she/her)

Ashley R. Hurst, JD, M.Div, MA (she/her)

Carrie McDermott, PhD, APRN, ACNS-BC (she/her)

Elizabeth Métraux (she/her)

Joy Miller, MSN, BS, RN, CPNP-PC, CHPPN (she/her)

Esther Golda Lozana Otis, BSN, RN, IBCLC (she/her)

Courtney M. Ott, DNP, MSN, BS, RN (she/her)

Kimberly Pate, DNP, RN, ACCNS-AG, PCCN, NE-BC, FCNS (she/her)

Arminda B. Perch, MBA, LCSW (she/her)

Erik Pérez, OTD, OTR (he/him)

Elizabeth A. (Lili) Powell, PhD (she/her)

Millie Sattler, DNP, MSN, RN, CCRN (she/her)

John Schorling, MD, MPH (he/him)

Ryan Thomas, BSN, RN, CCRN, NRP (he/him)

Special Note to Readers

Here at Sigma, we realize that language is constantly evolving. The meaning of a word often changes over time, some words become obsolete, and some terms that were once acceptable may become controversial or even offensive, depending on the context or circumstances. We have made every effort to make language choices that are inclusive and not offensive. Should you identify words in this book that you believe negatively impact a group or groups of people, please reach out to us at Publications@SigmaNursing.org.

Table of Contents

About the Authors...iii
Contributing Authors..v
Introduction..ix

section I — Fundamentals 1

1. The Fundamentals of Stress, Burnout, and Self-Care....... 2
2. The Fundamentals of Resilience, Growth, and Wisdom.... 6
3. Developing a Resilient Mindset Using Appreciative Practices 10

section II — The Mind of a Nurse 14

4. Self-Care, Communal Care, and Resilience Among Underrepresented Minoritized Nursing Professionals and Students 15
5. Self-Care for LGBTQIA+ Nursing Students 18
6. Racial Trauma and Healing.. 21
7. Narrative Practices.. 24
8. Self-Care and Systemic Change: What You Need to Know 27
9. Strengths-Based Self-Care: Good Enough, Strong Enough, Wise Enough 30

section III — The Body and Spirit of a Nurse............33

10. Reclaiming, Recalling, and Remembering: Spirituality and Self-Care 34
11. Sleep, Exercise, and Nutrition: Self-Care the Kaizen Way 37
12. Reflections on Self-Care and Your Clinical Practice 41

section IV — The Transition to Nursing Practice 44

13. Supportive Professional Relationships: Nurse Residency Programs, Preceptors, and Mentors............................ 45
14. Healthy Work Environment: How to Choose One for Your First Job 49
15. Self-Care for Humanitarian Aid Workers.................. 54

section V The Heart of a Nurse..........................57

- 16　Mattering: Creating a Rich Work Life.....................58
- 17　Integrating a Life That Works With a Life That Counts...61
- 18　Providing Compassionate Care and Addressing Unmet Social Needs Can Reduce Your Burnout...........64
- 19　Showing Up With Grit and Grace: How to Lead Under Pressure as a Nurse Clinician and Leader................67
- 20　Coaching Yourself When Things Are Hard...............70

Introduction

To ensure that we're all on the same page, let's revisit a few key points from the textbook:

- Self-care is not selfish. Nurses should be entitled, in fact expected, to care for themselves with the same creativity and compassion that they use to care for others.
- Nurses don't flourish simply by fostering the well-being of others. The nursing profession is inherently meaningful in that we care for patients and families during their most vulnerable moments. But meaningful work has its limits. A major thread throughout this book is that we don't want to be "the naked person offering someone their coat."
- Self-care is about the mind as much as it is about the body.
- Self-care is a lifelong *practice*, and it is best to begin the practice early, before facing the stressors of a hospital or other clinical setting. In general, student nurses face significantly more stress than their peers, increasing the importance and value of self-care practices during nursing school.
- Individual self-care practices do not let organizations off the hook. The importance of a healthy work environment cannot be overstated, and in this book, we offer help in selecting a healthy workplace and encourage readers to advocate for themselves and others.

Building a Self-Care Toolkit

This workbook, designed to be used with the textbook, will provide opportunities for you, the student nurse or new graduate nurse, to explore self-care behaviors that will help you deal with the big and small stressors you will encounter in your life or that you are encountering now. Our hope for you is that you will wholeheartedly "jump in" and explore both the practices outlined in this book and others that you encounter in this journey. Self-care has become an exciting field of study and practice, especially during the time of COVID-19 and other stressors that affect those of us who work in healthcare. There are so many resources to explore, and we have designed this workbook to encourage you to take advantage of as many of them as you can.

We encourage you to build your own self-care toolkit. Just like a carpentry toolkit or any toolkit, it will contain important items to help you be the best nurse (or carpenter) possible. The tools are essential to getting the job done. This self-care toolkit, instead of hammers, screwdrivers, and tape measures, will be a collection of a strategies, behaviors, and mindsets that will help you flourish in nursing.

To that end, we hope that you will try many of the practices shared here. Some will resonate with you immediately. Some will fit your lifestyle. Some will need modifying to suit your preferences. (Don't like writing down a gratitude list with paper and pen? Take photographs or use social media instead.) Some will just be completely wrong for you. Some might be intriguing to you, but maybe you'll decide to hold off and try them again in a few months or years. And even more exciting, there are dozens of ideas that we haven't thought of or tried yet. Explore practices on your own. If you are in a classroom or group setting, take advantage of your collective wisdom, and share your explorations with each other.

We cannot emphasize this enough: These practices take practice! So much of self-care is mental work, even more than the physical work of caring for your body. Our human brains are blessed with *neuroplasticity*, or the capacity to change. Just as you can build muscle tissue and train yourself in a physical skill such as bowling, roller skating, or playing the tuba, you can train your brain to react in new ways to stress and the challenges of your chosen profession.

When you have completed the readings in the textbook and the exercises in this workbook, we anticipate that you will have your own collection of self-care tools that you can practice regularly and rely on when you face challenges in your career and life. This self-care toolkit will help you build resilience to overcome a range of adversities, from daily annoyances to ongoing stressors to sudden loss or change.

The What-Why-Do-Reflect & Journal Format

The chapters in this workbook correspond to the chapters in the second edition of *Self-Care for New and Student Nurses*. The workbook exercises have been designed by the authors in consultation with our workbook chapter contributors. We encourage you to use the workbook as a complement to the textbook.

As nurses, we appreciate nothing more than order and structure. (Consider reporting structures, care plans, and checklists.) We take that approach with this workbook. We call it the *What-Why-Do-Reflect & Journal* format, and you will become very familiar with it as you move through this workbook. The *What-Why-Do-Reflect & Journal* structure provides a framework for exploring self-care behaviors by learning (or reviewing) what they are and why they matter for your well-being, trying them, and reflecting upon their usefulness to you in your life and clinical practice. By journaling, we encourage you to not only reflect on your progress but also keep track of which techniques feel right to you, which ones might need tweaking, and which ones might serve you well in the future.

section I
Fundamentals

1
The Fundamentals of Stress, Burnout, and Self-Care

—Natalie May

what

Read Chapter 1.

- What do we mean by the phrase "a naked person offering someone their shirt"?

- Describe the differences between stress, stressors, and burnout.

- List five stressors that nurses face in the workplace that are unique to healthcare and nursing.

    1. _____
    2. _____
    3. _____
    4. _____
    5. _____

- Why are new and early-career nurses more vulnerable to burnout and stress-related ill health than more experienced nurses?

- What barriers to self-care might you face as a practicing nurse?

why

- List three reasons a personal self-care practice is important for nurses.

    1. _____
    2. _____
    3. _____

- List three reasons a personal self-care practice is important *to you*.

    1. _____
    2. _____
    3. _____

do

Activity 1-1: My Current Self-Care Practice Inventory

- We are quite certain that you already engage in self-care practices, whether you label them as such or not. Think back over the past few years. What do you do to care for yourself when you feel stressed, anxious, or overwhelmed? Do you go for a run? Call a friend? Knit? Knock back a few beers? Do some online shopping? Write down all the activities that you turn to when you need to calm yourself.

- Once you have made this list, put a plus sign next to the activities that you think are helpful and that you would like to include in your self-care toolkit. Put a minus sign next to those that you might want to eliminate or modify, such as self-medicating with food or drink.

Activity 1-2: Self-Care Google Exploration

- This activity is included in the textbook. Google the terms "self-care" and "self-care practices." Expand your search if you're feeling especially ambitious or curious.

- Make a list of some of what pops up. You will find memes, posters, infographics, quotes, research articles, and more. Make a list, or a Pinterest board, of things that intrigue you or resonate with your personality and current self-care practices.

- Which concepts make you think, "I could get into this," or, "This makes sense to me"? What ideas intrigue you or make you want to learn more? These concepts might be your own personal entrées into the study and practice of self-care.

- As you are browsing the internet for self-care practices and ideas, try to categorize each practice into one of the following self-care and wellness categories: physical, mental, emotional, spiritual, intellectual, social, financial, and environmental. Some may fit into more than one category.

Activity 1-3: Try the Big Four

We end Chapter 1 with four of the fundamental self-care practices: staying hydrated; checking in with yourself and unclenching when you find tension in your body; taking deep, restorative breaths; and staying present. Begin to integrate these practices into your daily routine. Use whatever reminder system works best for you, whether it's alarms on your phone, post-it notes, or something else.

reflect & journal

- As you explore self-care practices in your Google search, try to imagine yourself engaging in some of these practices. Are you an athlete or an artist? Do you recoup your energy by being in nature? Is your highest priority staying connected with family and friends?
- What self-care practices would you like to learn more about and consider including in your self-care toolkit?
- Which of the Big Four practices (hydration, unclenching, breathing, being present) come most naturally to you? Which ones will take a little more work? Why?
- As you begin this journey, we want to caution you about comparing yourself to others. Comparing ourselves to others can often feel like a competition and can induce more stress and self-doubt. As you journal about your experiences with self-care, consider a different type of comparison. Compare yourself not to others, but to *you*. Observe the progress you have made. Celebrate your curiosity and willingness to try new things. Stick to it. Ask for help when you need it. Support and acknowledge the progress of others.

2
The Fundamentals of Resilience, Growth, and Wisdom

–Natalie May

what

Read Chapter 2.

- What do we mean by the term "resilience"?

- List three ways that your workplace can foster individual resilience.
    1. _____
    2. _____
    3. _____

- What are the four components of grit, another kind of resilience?
    1. _____
    2. _____
    3. _____
    4. _____

why

- Why is neuroplasticity important in our ability to become resilient?

- In this chapter, we present two nursing students, Nevin and Pat. Explain in your own words how these two students have learned to approach challenges. Which student do you most closely resemble? Why?

do

Activity 2-1: Foster Positive Emotions

One foundation of well-being is fostering positive emotions. Just as a steady diet of negativity will breed negativity, engaging in activities that make us feel good will help us feel good. Happiness and well-being researcher Barbara Frederickson (Cohn et al., 2009) identified 10 universal positive emotions that we ask you to explore here. For this activity, write down at least one activity or experience that gives rise to each emotion in you. For example, you might feel awe when you see a hawk fly overhead. Perhaps you feel inspiration when you observe an experienced nurse perform a difficult procedure. After identifying what creates positive emotions, the next step is to be intentional about experiencing them. If calling your best friend generates feelings of love, call your best friend more often. If a particular song makes you feel joyful, listen to that song!

Emotion	Activity
Joy	
Gratitude	
Serenity	
Interest	
Hope	
Pride	
Amusement	
Inspiration	
Awe	
Love	

Activity 2-2: Savor the Moment

Rick Hanson (2018) argues that we must "sit with" positive emotions to rewire our brains for resilience. In Chapter 2, we provided a hypothetical list of daily opportunities to savor positive emotions. For at least one day, be very intentional about savoring positive moments, from the moment you wake up until you fall asleep at night. Write down as many of these moments as possible. After this one-day exercise, remind yourself to continue savoring positive emotions.

reflect & journal

- How will you be able to maintain this practice of fostering positive emotions and savoring them once you are in clinical practice? What techniques and strategies can you use to help build these activities into your daily and weekly routine?

- We all know someone, either personally or from the news or history books, who has overcome extreme adversity and grown wiser as a result of their experience. In the textbook, we include Congressman John Lewis, Malala Yousafzai, and the Marjorie Stoneman Douglas High School students as examples of individuals who were able to transform their pain into wisdom. Who do you know that you would consider wise? Why do you consider them to be wise? What qualities do they exhibit? Did they overcome adversity as part of their journey to wisdom?

- How does it feel to be intentional about fostering and savoring positive emotions? Is this a new experience for you? Is it something that you can continue to do? Why or why not?

- You are capable. You are strong. You are wise. You will become more able, strong, and wise as you learn and grow. Say it aloud to yourself: "I am capable. I am strong. I am wise." Believe it.

references

Cohn, M. A., Fredrickson, B. L., Brown, S. L., Mikels, J. A., & Conway, A. M. (2009). Happiness unpacked: Positive emotions increase life satisfaction by building resilience. *Emotion, 9*(3), 361–368. https://doi.org/10.1037/a0015952

Hanson, R. (2018). *Resilient: How to grow an unshakable core of calm, strength, and happiness.* Harmony Books.

3
Developing a Resilient Mindset Using Appreciative Practices

–Natalie May & Julie Haizlip

what

Read Chapter 3.

- What is the negativity bias? Give some examples of this bias in your own life.

- What are some of the well-being benefits of positive activities?

- Explain two of the theoretical principles (constructionist, poetic, positive, simultaneity, anticipatory) of Appreciative Inquiry in your own words.

why

In this chapter, the authors discuss the importance of "choosing our focus." Explain what this entails and why it matters. (You may want to refer back to the Nevin and Pat examples in Chapter 2.)

do

Activity 3-1: Choose Language With Care

As the authors explain, language creates our reality. Observe the choices that people make with language. How does naming something a certain way change the words' impact? Pay attention to your own language choices. Did you learn to use certain words in your childhood that seem problematic today?

Activity 3-2: Reframing

What we choose to focus on becomes our fate (Whitney & Trosten-Bloom, 2003). *Reframing* is the capacity to intentionally explore new ways of seeing to experience the best of what is. Think of something that is annoying, sad, disappointing, or challenging. Now reframe this situation to find the best of what is. For example, you may have a long walk to your campus or hospital. You could reframe this by realizing that the walk is an opportunity for exercise, time to listen to music, or a chance to prepare for or decompress from your day.

Activity 3-3: Gratitude Practice

A growing body of research finds that a simple gratitude practice can improve well-being among nurses and other healthcare workers (Sexton & Adair, 2019). Commit to taking time at the end of each day to write down three good things that happened to you during the day. These can be exciting events such as acing an exam or receiving a job offer, but most likely, they will be more humble moments. You might appreciate a delicious meal, an unexpected connection with a friend, a nap, or a sunny day.

You may choose to write your three good things in a small notebook, on your phone, or on your laptop. The most important thing is to do it regularly for at least 10 days. You will begin to notice that throughout the day, your attention and thoughts will be drawn toward those good things around you and away from those things that produce negative feelings.

If you would like to take this exercise a step further, pick one good thing each day and reflect on the people and events that made that good thing possible. For example, if you are grateful for a hot cup of coffee, think about the barista who made it to work that day and the workers who manufactured the cups; you will increase your sense of connection with the world around you.

Activity 3-4: Positivity Portfolio

A *positivity portfolio* is a collection of objects, words, or photos that stirs positive emotions in the viewer or reader. Positivity portfolios are more common than we realize. A collection of photos, plants, and seashells on someone's desk is a positivity portfolio. Refrigerator magnets that remind a family of their travels together is a positivity portfolio. A collection of favorite quotes and a laptop or water bottle covered in stickers are positivity portfolios. A playlist can be a positivity portfolio. Create your own portfolio in any way you choose. All that matters is that you create a collection of items that make you feel a positive emotion, such as happiness, contentment, or peace.

Activity 3-5: Vision Board

We move toward the image of the future that we hold in our heads, and the more positive that vision, the more positive our future. Remember the story of Ryan Speedo Green, the young man who saw his first opera at the Met and visualized himself performing at that same stage someday. Creating positive visions of our future is a remarkably powerful tool.

To create a vision board, gather a stack of old magazines, scissors, a piece of cardstock or cardboard, and a glue stick. Give yourself at least an hour (set a timer) to flip through the magazines and cut out photos and words that represent the future you are seeking. Relax. What dreams do you have for yourself? (This exercise can be done for the upcoming year or a longer time frame, whichever seems best to you.) Cut and glue the pictures to your cardstock and keep the collage somewhere you can see it regularly.

Activity 3-6: Vision Board, With No Glue

Are you trying to make a difficult decision about your future? Is there something you desire, but you are having trouble achieving it? Create a quiet space and give yourself at least a half hour to do this activity. Visualize your life one year from now. What does it look like? The power is in the details. Imagine yourself waking up in the morning. Where are you? What do you eat for breakfast? Is someone with you, or are you alone? Go through your entire day in this future life, focusing on your work, your friends, the activities of your day. *Remember—details, details, details.* Pay attention to how you feel. On a piece of paper, write down as many details as you can remember.

reflect & journal

- We hope this chapter gave you a lot of ideas and food for thought. Which activities were the most helpful? Were any so compelling that you think you could include them in your self-care toolkit?
- "Our focus is our fate." Spend a few moments writing about your own focus and how it affects your well-being in the short and long term.

references

Sexton, J. B., & Adair, K. C. (2019). Forty-five good things: A prospective pilot study of the Three Good Things well-being intervention in the USA for healthcare worker emotional exhaustion, depression, work-life balance and happiness. *BMJ Open, 9*(3), e022695. https://doi.org/10.1136/bmjopen-2018-022695

Whitney, D., & Trosten-Bloom, A. (2003). *The power of appreciative inquiry: A practical guide to positive change.* Berrett-Koehler Publishers, Inc.

section II
The Mind of a Nurse

4
Self-Care, Communal Care, and Resilience Among Underrepresented Minoritized Nursing Professionals and Students

—Ebru Çayir

what

Read Chapter 4.

- Describe at least five unique challenges underrepresented minority (URM) nurses face.

    1. _____
    2. _____
    3. _____
    4. _____
    5. _____

- The author states, "Nurses' experiences of emotional labor are not only gendered but also racialized." Explain what she means by this.

- What unique barriers to self-care do URM nurses face?

why

- Why is communal care a potentially more effective strategy for well-being than self-care?

do

Activity 4-1: Responding to Discriminatory Behavior: Individuals

Have you experienced or observed racial or ethnic identity-based discriminative experiences during your training? If so, what was your response or the response of others? If possible, gather in a group of four to five peers, establish expectations for students to safely share their experiences, and begin this conversation. Give yourselves time to make sure that all voices are heard.

Activity 4-2: Responding to Discriminatory Behavior: Healthcare Institutions

Reflect on and discuss with your peers how healthcare institutions can address the issues URM nursing professionals and students experience. What types of resources are available in your institution that might help address these issues? Are there any structural and policy changes you would like to see?

Generate a list of policy and health system changes your team envisions that would build equity, inclusion, and diversity into your school or workplace.

reflect & journal

- Think about examples of communal care in your own life and how they have had an impact on your well-being. Now consider ways that communal care and similar well-being benefits can be cultivated in healthcare organizations. What would our healthcare organizations look like, and in what ways would they focus on diversity, inclusion, and equity?

- Dr. Çayir selected this quote by Maya Angelou to open her chapter: "My mission in life is not merely to survive, but to thrive; and to do so with some passion, some compassion, some humor, and some style." Imagine yourself in your role as a nurse. In what ways will you embody these qualities—passion, compassion, humor, and style—in your work and life?

5
Self-Care for LGBTQIA+ Nursing Students

–Kim Acquaviva

what

Read Chapter 5.

- List the additional stressors faced by LGBTQIA+ nursing students.

- Given these additional stressors, self-care strategies are vitally important for the LGBTQIA+ nursing student. Describe the four LGBTQIA+–specific self-care strategies that the author suggests in this chapter.

    1. _____
    2. _____
    3. _____
    4. _____

why

This chapter opens with the famous quote by Audre Lorde: "Caring for myself is not self-indulgence, it is self-preservation, and that is an act of political warfare" (Lorde, 1988, p. 205). Why is caring for oneself an act of political warfare?

do

Activity 5-1: The Importance of Being Seen

If you identify as LGBTQIA+, how did it feel reading a chapter that was written in a voice that was clearly speaking to you? Think of times in your life when you have felt seen. What specific behaviors on the part of others make you feel this way?

If you identify as heterosexual and cisgender, how did it feel reading a chapter that was written in a voice that was clearly speaking to someone other than you? In what ways did the author express her compassion and understanding for her readers? Think of times in your life when you have felt seen for who you truly are. What specific behaviors on the part of others make you feel this way?

reflect & journal

- In what ways can you be more intentional about helping others feel truly seen by you?
- Identity is complex—LGBTQIA+ nursing students aren't *just* LGBTQIA+. They hold other identities simultaneously: Black, Latinx, Indigenous/Native, Jewish, Christian, Muslim, atheist, first-generation college student, and so on. LGBTQIA+ nursing students may also be persons with disabilities or persons for whom English is the second language they learned.
- What identities do you hold? How do you care for each of those identities?

references

Lorde, A. (1988). *A burst of light: And other essays.* Courier Dover Publications.

6
Racial Trauma and Healing

–Arminda Perch

what

Read Chapter 6.

- Explain what defines a trauma or traumatic event.

- What are some of the responses individuals have to trauma?

- What is vicarious trauma?

- Explain race-based stress and trauma and its impact on those who experience it.

- What are the three central tasks required for recovery of racial trauma? What does each entail?
    1. _____
    2. _____
    3. _____

why

What is the goal of recovery from racial trauma?

do

Activity 6-1: Learn More About Racial Trauma and Healing

If you have not experienced racial trauma yourself, some of the material in this chapter may have been new to you. You could take this as an invitation to learn more about the experiences of your peers or co-workers. If you are reading this text in a course, ask if the minoritized students would be comfortable talking about their experiences with racial trauma. It is important to create a safe space for sharing these stories. Other students should listen respectfully and ask curious questions if appropriate. If this sharing isn't an option, there are countless books, movies, and podcasts that can help us learn more about the experiences of others in our communities.

What resources are available to students in your school who have experienced racial trauma?

Activity 6-2: Use the Tools

In this chapter, the author offers many concrete steps an individual can take to move toward healing. They are presented in the context of racial trauma and healing. If you are someone who has experienced racial trauma, what steps might you take today to begin your healing journey?

If you have not personally experienced racial trauma, how might the steps be helpful in coping with challenges in your own life?

reflect & journal

How has reading this chapter shifted your perspective and changed how you might interact with your peers and future patients?

7
Narrative Practices

–Tim Cunningham

what

Read Chapter 7.

- This chapter is about *paying attention*. How can narrative practices, and other activities that foster deep awareness, help you become a better clinician?

- Describe the three levels of resonance, or caring: sympathetic, empathetic, and compassionate.

    1. _____
    2. _____
    3. _____

why

In considering our ability to reflect, refract, and deflect emotions, why is awareness of this phenomenon so important to nurses? What examples can you provide?

do

Activity 7-1: Visual Arts

In groups of three or four, collectively select a famous painting or sculpture. You may consider browsing websites of a local art museum to find images on the web. Once you find the image, designate one person in the group to prompt discussion questions about the image. (This exercise may certainly be done on your own, but it is an excellent group activity.) Here is a list of museum websites:

- **The Tate Modern:** https://www.tate.org.uk
- **The Metropolitan Museum of Art:** https://www.metmuseum.org
- **Museo Botero:** https://www.banrepcultural.org/bogota/museo-botero
- **The National Bardo Museum:** http://www.bardomuseum.tn

- Tokyo National Museum: https://www.tnm.jp/?lang=en
- National Museum Australia: https://www.nma.gov.au

Ask the following questions of the group, and allow time for everyone to respond.

1. What comes to mind first when you see this image?
2. What is the first feeling (if any) that comes up for you?
3. Look closely now at the textures of the image. What do you see?
4. Look closely now at the colors in the image. What do you see?
5. What do you think the artist was trying to say with this piece of work?
6. If you could meet the artist right now, what would you tell them about this work?

Activity 7-2: Capturing Your Own Experience in Art

Think of a patient encounter or healthcare experience that had meaning to you. Select an art form—prose or poetry writing, painting, drawing, collage, music, photography—and convey your experience of this encounter. Relax and enjoy this process. There is no right or wrong, good or bad.

reflect & journal

- In this chapter, the author writes, "That calling [to become a nurse] is at the core of our lived experience. Uniquely ours, lived experience is an important aspect of our lives to examine because, from it, we will know ourselves better. In knowing ourselves better, we'll better understand our own individual and critical self-care needs." Write about your calling to become a nurse. What is your story?
- Select a narrative of health, illness, or healing to read. You may choose one of the books included in this chapter (e.g., *Violation*, *When Breath Becomes Air*, *Fun Home*) or choose one of the many others that have been written. If an entire book feels daunting, select an essay or short story. Use the narrative practice skills we have discussed to reflect on the work you chose. How did the work make you feel? How did it change you? What did it convey about the author and their experience of health, illness, or healing?

8
Self-Care and Systemic Change: What You Need to Know

–Ashley Hurst

what

Read Chapter 8.

- There are pitfalls to focusing on individual self-care above all else. What are the author's concerns about this?

- Explain moral distress in your own words. Provide at least one example.

- The author writes, "Pairing self-care practices with advocacy empowers nurses to change systems that are not promoting health for all." What is the #selfcare movement? Why is it potentially harmful for true well-being?

why

Why is the "mythology of heroic, self-sacrificing women who cared for the sick" problematic for the well-being of today's nurses?

do

Activity 8-1: The Mythology of Nursing

This chapter links the origin myths and stereotypes of nursing to many of the underlying systemic issues in healthcare today. Dig a little deeper into this notion of potentially harmful perceptions of nursing and nurses. What misperceptions have you personally encountered? What stereotypes did you grow up with? Have these stereotypical images changed since you've become a nursing student?

Activity 8-2: #selfcare

In Chapter 1, we invited you to do a Google search of self-care practices. Our goal was to give you a broad sense of the self-care activities and options available to you as you begin this journey. We suggested that you view your search results through a personal lens: What practices were appealing to you? Which were you curious to learn more about? Now we invite you to revisit your Google search, or do another one, and look at the search results through the #selfcare lens. Which create unrealistic expectations? Which may not be based in good science? Which promote unhelpful stereotypes? Which are actually ridiculous? Which might be harmful?

reflect & journal

Imagine yourself in an unhealthy work environment. (We hope this doesn't happen to you.) What would you do in that situation? What options might you have?

It is discouraging to think that your workplace may not prioritize the well-being of its employees. As we wrote in the editors' introduction to the textbook chapter, there is a tension between self-care and institutional responsibility. Give yourself some time and space to reflect and write on this difficult issue.

9
Strengths-Based Self-Care: Good Enough, Strong Enough, Wise Enough

–Tim Cunningham

what

Read Chapter 9.

- What is the "victim narrative"? How can it be detrimental to well-being?

- Explain posttraumatic growth (PTG) in your own words.

- What are the five elements of PTG?
    1. _____
    2. _____
    3. _____
    4. _____
    5. _____

- List the five aspects of high emotional intelligence.
    1. _____
    2. _____
    3. _____
    4. _____
    5. _____

why

Why might "not taking it personally" be one of the most valuable tools in your self-care toolkit?

do

Activity 9-1: Growth From Trauma

Take some time to read about a person you admire. They could be a civil rights or political leader, community advocate, artist, scientist, businessperson, or celebrity. You might choose a nurse, friend, or loved one. As you learn about this person, consider any trauma that they experienced. How did that trauma lead to transformation and growth? What strengths did they draw on to help them navigate the traumatic event?

Activity 9-2: Inherent Strengths Inventory

This chapter contends that we all have inherent strengths, and we can build on these strengths as a form of self-care. In other words, we don't have to begin from scratch, and we don't have to learn everything anew. We each have qualities and characteristics that will help us navigate adversity, grow, and maintain our well-being. We invite you to create your own strengths inventory. Consider traits that are included in this chapter, but we encourage you to expand your view to include other qualities as well.

reflect & journal

How have you moved through adversity or trauma in your life? How did that experience transform you, in good ways and bad?

section III
The Body and Spirit of a Nurse

10
Reclaiming, Recalling, and Remembering: Spirituality and Self-Care

–Robin Brown-Haithcoa

what

Read Chapter 10.

- How does this author define "spirituality"?

- What does the author mean by "vocation"?

- Describe the term "paradoxical thinking" and give three examples.

    1. _____
    2. _____
    3. _____

why

Why is it important to acknowledge and talk about "our true selves"?

do

Activity 10-1: Defining a Belief System

Consider your own belief system, or your guiding principles, and write answers to the following questions.

- Who, or what, encouraged you to believe as you do? What in your own life narrative has led you to these beliefs?
- Are your beliefs based on a traditional spiritual practice or something else?
- What specifically are your guiding principles?

- How do your guiding principles affect your daily living? (This could include decision-making, self-care, or simply the way you show up in the world.)
- How do you nurture your spiritual practice or belief system?
- Tell a story about a time that your spiritual practice allowed you to move through a challenging time to a place of peace, compassion, love, or hope.

reflect & journal

- How will your values or beliefs guide your professional role as a nurse?
- The author includes a quote by Parker Palmer who says we will find our vocation by accepting the "treasure of true self" we already possess. He encourages us to listen for and nurture that true self. Do you think you know who your true self is?

11
Sleep, Exercise, and Nutrition: Self-Care the Kaizen Way

–Tim Cunningham

what

Read Chapter 11.

- Explain the philosophy of Kaizen. How does it relate to a self-care practice?

- List five nonpharmacological sleep aids.

    1. _____
    2. _____
    3. _____
    4. _____
    5. _____

- What are some of the well-being benefits of exercise? Of sexual activity?

- What are the barriers to healthy, nutritious eating faced by many nurses? (You may want to refer to Chapter 1 in the textbook as well.)

why

There are so many voices (experts and otherwise) telling us what to eat to maintain good health. In determining your own nutrition choices, who is the most important expert and why?

do

Activity 11-1: The Sleep-Exercise-Nutrition Triangle

This is an exercise to foster awareness of the connection between the three sides of the sleep-exercise-nutrition triangle and to help you pay attention to your own physical well-being. For seven days, keep track of your sleep, physical activity, and nutrition with simple +, –, or = signs. + indicates that you feel you did well in caring for yourself and meeting your physical needs; – indicates that you think you could have done better; and = indicates you aren't sure, or you are simply satisfied but not impressed. If you'd prefer, you may provide more detailed information in your chart, but our goal is to keep things simple.

Day	Sleep	Exercise	Nutrition	Notes
Example	+	–	=	Pouring rain; couldn't run Ate OK; didn't snack
1				
2				
3				
4				
5				
6				
7				

After seven days, can you see any patterns? If you had poor sleep on certain days, did exercise and nutrition suffer on those days, too? Are you consistently getting enough sleep but not enough exercise? Describe all the patterns that you notice. What factors had an impact on your physical self-care during this week?

Activity 11-2: Paying Attention

As you went through the week charting your physical self-care, we expect that you may have been paying close attention to your body in a new way. What kinds of things did you notice? What messages did your body send you? For example, how did your body feel after drinking beverages that contain sugar, caffeine, or alcohol?

Activity 11-3: The Kaizen Way

Consider what you learned this week using a Kaizen mindset. Where do you see opportunities for small steps that might result in change? Think about the sleep-exercise-nutrition triad, and identify one small change you can make. Commit to it for 10 days. We offer a few suggestions to get you thinking. Of course, refer to the *Self-Care* textbook and other sources for more ideas.

- Take the stairs instead of using the elevator.
- Turn off all screens 15 minutes before you lie down to sleep.
- Eat vegetarian for one meal a day.
- Pack healthy snacks—fruit, sugar-free yogurt, trail mix—in your backpack.
- Park farther away and walk.
- Use a sleep app to help you fall asleep.
- Eat one meal each day slowly and mindfully.
- Drink a glass of water first thing in the morning.

If this exercise resonates with you, consider adding one small change to the mix each week. Notice what larger changes begin to happen in your life.

reflect & journal

- What if, in this moment, you are good enough? We can say with surety that you *are* good enough. This chapter is not about being good or bad but about caring for yourself, especially your physical self. This chapter is about paying attention to your body so that you can respond to its needs. If your body needs something (more sleep, more movement, better fuel), you can make those changes slowly, one at a time.
- Write down all the reasons that you want to care for your body.

12
Reflections on Self-Care and Your Clinical Practice

—Joy Miller

what

Read Chapter 12.

- How does this author create in-the-moment self-care opportunities in the middle of a busy clinical practice?

- What is a transition ritual?

- What does the author mean when she writes about "set an intention" or "intention setting"?

why

Why does the author sometimes cringe when she looks back on her early days as a nurse?

do

Activity 12-1: Transition Rituals

The chapter author uses journaling as a transition activity before and after her shifts. We know other nurses who use prayer, exercise, music, or meditation to help them prepare or decompress. What transition rituals have you used in the past, even if you didn't name them as such? Try at least one transition ritual this week as you come and go to school or your clinical rotations.

Activity 12-2: To-Be-Joyful (*Not* a To-Do) List

In a chapter sidebar, Jennifer shares ways that she cares for herself on her days off. One way is to make a list of activities; the list makes her feel productive and allows her to intentionally focus on self-care. "This list keeps me reminded of activities outside of work that help me de-stress and stay organized. As I cross these tasks off my list, I earn my sense of productivity and feel ready to give back to others around me."

Imagine that you have all the time in the world to do things that make you happy. Write a list of these activities.

Activity 12-3: Frames of Reference

Review the author's description of her frames of reference, her guiding principles for showing up as a nurse. What frames of reference do you think would serve you well in your clinical practice? How do they build on the guiding principles that you live by today?

reflect & journal

- The textbook focuses a lot of attention on physical self-awareness—noticing when you are tense, tired, thirsty, and more. This chapter approaches self-awareness from a different perspective. What kind of self-awareness makes the author the kind of nurse that she is?
- We especially love the author's description of Tonglen practice and how she uses the practice to foster loving-kindness toward those she encounters in her practice. We encourage you to learn more about this practice as a way to "set your intentions" toward your patients.
- The chapter author closes by writing about boundaries as a form of self-care. What are your boundaries in your life today? What additional boundaries would you like to establish?

section IV
The Transition to Nursing Practice

13
Supportive Professional Relationships: Nurse Residency Programs, Preceptors, and Mentors

–Carrie McDermott & Millie Sattler

what

Read Chapter 13.

- List the seven major challenges that newly licensed registered nurses face.

    1. _____
    2. _____
    3. _____
    4. _____
    5. _____
    6. _____
    7. _____

- What are the goals of transition-to-practice nurse residency programs?

- Describe the benefits of having a mentor.

- A nurse mentor can serve as a coach, counselor, confidant, encourager, friend, visionary, and resource. What roles should a mentor *not* embrace?

13 Supportive Professional Relationships: Nurse Residency Programs, Preceptors, and Mentors

why

Why should nurses and mentors set specific goals, and what might they entail?

do

Activity 13-1: Investigate NRPs

Spend some time researching hospitals or health systems and their nurse residency programs (NRPs). Do they meet all the criteria outlined in this chapter, such as being nine to 12 months long, having an evidence-based curriculum, and so on? Are they accredited by the Commission on Collegiate Nursing Education or the American Nurses Credentialing Center? Do they offer evidence-based practice projects? (Review the NRP checklist at the end of the chapter.)

Activity 13-2: S.M.A.R.T. Goal Setting

Goal setting is an important part of the mentoring experience for both the mentee and the mentor. But what is a good goal? What are some criteria by which you can assess the strength of a goal? One way to structure goals is by using the S.M.A.R.T. goal approach. S.M.A.R.T. stands for Specific, Measurable, Achievable, Relevant, and Time-based. Consider one goal for yourself that you can achieve this month. It can be anything related to school, work, home, or self-care. In the following table, complete a S.M.A.R.T. diagram for your goal. Enter the name of your goal and generate the S.M.A.R.T. steps you will take to achieve it. Once you write this out, take steps toward completing that goal.

Name of Goal:	Responses:
Specific: Write out details about what this goal entails.	
Measurable: Write out exactly how you will measure accomplishment of this goal.	
Achievable: Is this goal achievable? How do you know? What have you achieved before this point that will help you know you can reach this one?	
Relevant: Write how this goal aligns with who you are, your personal beliefs, and your larger goals in life.	
Time-based: What is the realistic time frame during which you can begin to work on this goal and when you plan to achieve it? Are there milestones or checkpoints along the way that you can list to hit while you are achieving this goal?	

reflect & journal

- It's not all about the mentor. It is also the mentee's responsibility to collaborate effectively with the mentor and develop a trusting relationship. Zachary (2012) came up with nine essential mentee skills, listed next. Consider your own skills for each of these areas. Where are your strengths, and where might you need some improvement? What might you do to strengthen some of these skills?

    1. Ability to receive and give feedback
    2. Self-directed
    3. Open communicator
    4. Taking initiative
    5. Valuing self-reflection
    6. Ability to listen
    7. Ability to follow through
    8. Relationship building
    9. Ability to set goals

- In today's fast-paced "gig economy," some say that mentoring in nursing may be a dying art. How can you serve as a mentor to others today and in the future? Perhaps you are already serving in a mentoring role, either formal or informal. How can you reignite the art of mentoring?

reference

Zachary, L. J. (2012). *The mentor's guide* (2nd ed.). Jossey-Bass.

14
Healthy Work Environment: How to Choose One for Your First Job

–Dorrie K. Fontaine

what

Read Chapter 14.

- List the six standards for establishing and sustaining a healthy work environment (HWE).

    1. _____
    2. _____
    3. _____
    4. _____
    5. _____
    6. _____

- "Skilled communication" is a broad standard that includes a range of important topics. List at least five aspects of skilled communication in an HWE.

    1. _____
    2. _____
    3. _____
    4. _____
    5. _____

- What distinguishes the Daisy Award as a meaningful form of recognition for nurses?

why

Why are some environments healthier than others? What factors have you observed in clinical settings that have led you to say, "This would be a good place to work," or, "This is not a place I would like to work"?

do

Activity 14-1: Identifying Priorities for Your First Job

Reflect on the priorities you might consider when choosing your first job in nursing. Rank the following seven criteria on level of importance from 1 to 7, where 1 has the highest importance to you and 7 has the lowest, at least in the early stages of your career. Use the table to rank these items and briefly describe your reasoning or considerations for each ranking. We have included additional rows for you to add other priorities, if needed.

Priority	Rank (1–7)	Reasons for Ranking/Factors to Consider
Geographic location		
Specialty		
Reputation of organization		
Proximity to family and friends		
Availability or quality of a nurse residency program		
Type of hospital: teaching vs. community or private		
"Feel"/support of the work environment		

Activity 14-2: Rocking the Interview

One strategy to land that first exciting position in your top hospital and unit is to shine in the interview. Following are several questions to consider. As you read through the list, consider what to add and perhaps put a star next to the ones that underscore your most important values and priorities. We have used the HWE standards to frame these as well as Jennifer Hargreaves and Christine Pabico's 2020 article, "How to Choose Your First Nursing Job Wisely." They acknowledge that nurse leaders will carefully interview you to make sure you are the right fit. You should be doing the same interviewing: Is this hospital the right fit for you? Their suggestions come from the American Nurses Credentialing Center Pathway to Excellence Interview Tool (Hargreaves & Pabico, 2020).

Interview Questions to Ask

1. Does your organization use the AACN Standards for an HWE? (Bring a copy to the interview.)
2. Is there Magnet® designation? Beacon units?
3. How long is the nurse residency program? What are the components?
4. Describe the orientation program. Is there a potential to increase it if needed?
5. What are the nurse turnover/retention rate and nurse vacancy rates for the past two years?
6. What do nurses state as their reason for leaving?
7. Are there programs for nursing staff development such as Crucial Conversations, patient safety, and clinical topics? Are these programs interprofessional, including physicians and other disciplines?
8. Describe the shared governance program and the committees where staff nurses are engaged.
9. What happens when there is conflict or disrespect? Are there policies in place based upon the ANA recommendations?
10. How visible is the nurse manager on the unit? Do they wear scrubs, at least some of the time?
11. What are the biggest challenges nurses face each day? How is the nurse staffing determined? Has there been turnover in the nursing leadership recently?
12. Describe the clinical ladder. Are there awards for nurses? Is the hospital signed on to provide the Daisy Award to nurses?
13. What are the hospital's most notable successes?
14. Describe the programs for nurse well-being.

reflect & journal

- Choosing your first nursing job probably feels stressful, but we hope this chapter has helped you feel a little less so. What are your concerns, fears, and worries about your first job? What elements of your first work environment might alleviate some of those concerns?

- This might be a good time to encourage you to reflect on all the accomplishments you have already achieved, all the challenges you have met with grace and energy, and the many skills you have mastered. Set a timer for 10 minutes and make a list of all you are proud of about yourself. Write quickly, and do not think too much. Just write.

- The importance of "meaningful recognition" came to the fore during the COVID-19 pandemic. Citizens applauded healthcare workers during shift changes. We left our Christmas lights up through the winter to acknowledge their service. Many were celebrated as "heroes." Yet in many hospitals, nurses felt the sting of "*unmeaningful* recognition," such as free pizzas, buttons, or T-shirts. We often heard nurses say something like, "Don't tell me I'm a hero. Just wear your damn mask." What really *is* meaningful recognition? Does it depend on the circumstances? On the individual nurse? What meaningful recognition have you received or would you like to receive?

reference

Hargreaves, J., & Pabico, C. (2020). How to choose your first nursing job wisely. *American Nurse Journal, 15*(5), 30–31.

15
Self-Care for Humanitarian Aid Workers

—Tim Cunningham

what

Read Chapter 15.

- What are the global and humanitarian crises that give rise to the need to deploy healthcare workers?

- What are the basic skills needed for nursing work in humanitarian settings?

- What are the five forms of self-care the author and his colleagues used to care for themselves while helping Ebola victims?

    1. _____
    2. _____
    3. _____
    4. _____
    5. _____

why

Why is self-care even more important for humanitarian aid workers than traditional healthcare workers? What additional stressors do they face?

do

Activity 15-1: Fictional and Nonfictional Healthcare Workers

Read, or reread, a book about healthcare workers in challenging circumstances. We offer a few wonderful choices to get you started. As you read, consider how self-care factors into the subject's work, if at all.

> *The Plague*, by Albert Camus
>
> *Cutting for Stone*, by Abraham Verghese
>
> *The Shift*, by Theresa Brown
>
> *Being Mortal*, by Atul Gawande
>
> *Mountains Beyond Mountains*, by Tracey Kidder

Activity 15-2: Interview Humanitarian or Pandemic Workers

Interview a student, a nurse peer, or a nursing professor who has worked in a humanitarian setting or during the AIDS epidemic of the 1980s and 1990s. You may also want to interview a nurse who worked during the COVID-19 pandemic. Ask them to describe the work they did and what motivated them to care for their patients. What challenges did they face? How did they take care of themselves? How did they balance their work with the concerns of their families and loved ones?

Activity 15-3: Blogging

We have encouraged you to reflect on your experiences with journal writing, but have you considered sharing your thoughts with others? Many humanitarian workers write online blogs so they can share their experience with others, to feel heard, and with the hope of creating change. Sharing personal narratives can be an opportunity for others, not only humanitarian nurses, to have their voices heard. Consider starting now. As a nursing student or early career nurse, what experiences would be of interest to others? What universal lessons and wisdom are you gaining that you could share with others? Determine your audience and your unique perspective and write a blog post. You might also consider writing an editorial; your school of nursing probably has a communications director who would be willing to help you find a publication "home" for it.

reflect & journal

- This chapter reminds us that self-care must be fluid and flexible, not only in humanitarian settings but also in more traditional healthcare environments. When have you been successful in staying flexible during difficult situations? How did that flexibility benefit your well-being?

- Humor has been an important aspect of self-care for this author and others in humanitarian settings. But humor can be dark, and it can diminish those around us. This is especially fraught in healthcare settings. Have you experienced a time when you or others were using humor at other people's expense?

section V
The Heart of a Nurse

16
Mattering: Creating a Rich Work Life

—Julie Haizlip

what

Read Chapter 16.

- Mattering is a fascinating concept and one you probably haven't studied before. What are the four domains of interpersonal mattering?

    1. _____
    2. _____
    3. _____
    4. _____

- Explain the differences between interpersonal mattering and societal mattering.

- In the study conducted by the author, what were the opportunities for nurses to feel like they mattered at work?

why

- Why is mattering an important concept in the context of nursing education and training? Think not only of "traditional" nursing students but students who tend to be marginalized.

- How does a sense of mattering factor into a nurse's sense of well-being and resilience?

do

Activity 16-1: When Do I Matter?

Take a moment to think about your experience as a nursing student. Who or what has made you feel like you matter? When have you felt seen or heard? How have you, or could you have, added value? Write or tell the story of a time when you felt like you mattered.

Activity 16-2: Mattering and Patient Care

Clinicals also provide an opportunity to spend a few extra minutes with a patient. What can you learn about that patient as a person? Perhaps they could share with you what their experience has been with the illness or issue that brought them to the hospital or clinic. How is this experience affecting their life? What do they value most about the care their nurses provide? What advice would they have for you as a future nurse? Asking questions and taking the time to listen to the answers provides a valuable service to anyone but is particularly important if a person is alone, confused, scared, or uncomfortable. You have the potential to make that person feel seen and heard and to show them that they matter. You can add value by helping that individual feel valued. You may also learn something that has been overlooked or not considered by the team caring for that person and can serve everyone involved by bringing that something to light.

Activity 16-3: Do Students Matter?

Clinical instructors and preceptors choose to work with student nurses because they are invested in your education. In addition to learning about physical assessment, medications, and the art of caring for another person, take a moment to learn something about your preceptor. Why did they choose nursing? What do they enjoy most about working with students? What is the most important thing they do in a day's work? Can your preceptor tell you about a time when they felt like they mattered? The answers to these questions will provide you with valuable insight into the profession of nursing and may provide a much-needed boost for your preceptor. We hope you will find that students play an important role in preceptors' sense of mattering.

reflect & journal

- The chapter ends by pointing out that there will be times you won't receive the feedback or recognition reminding you that you matter. What will you do to foster your own sense of mattering?
- How can you help others feel as if they matter? This can include fellow students, patients, and colleagues.

17
Integrating a Life That Works With a Life That Counts

—Dorrie K. Fontaine

what

Read Chapter 17.

- Describe David Whyte's "three marriages" metaphor.

- List three ways to foster authenticity in your personal and work relationships.

    1. _____
    2. _____
    3. _____

- The chapter offers seven specific strategies for creating and maintaining an integrated life. What are they?

    1. _____
    2. _____
    3. _____
    4. _____
    5. _____
    6. _____
    7. _____

why

Why does the author prefer the term "work-life integration" over "work-life balance"?

do

Activity 17-1: Pebble in Your Shoe

The author talks about the Joy in Work project that revealed weekend and evening emails were a "pebble in the shoe" of her faculty. To increase joy in the workplace, the school simply stopped weekend and evening emails, as well as the expectation that these off-hours emails must be answered.

Consider a simple change you could make that could greatly improve your happiness and joy. Make that change and see what happens when you no longer have that pebble in your shoe.

Activity 17-2: Eavesdropping

The first step in creating an integrated life is "knowing yourself" so that you will be free and able to reveal yourself to others. Give yourself time and space (at least 30 minutes) to imagine that it's your nursing school graduation celebration. All the most important people in your life are in attendance—family, friends, teachers, colleagues, patients, and more. You notice a group of them talking animatedly, smiling, and nodding. They are talking about how much they love and care about you and why. They share why they admire you, what they value most about you, and how you have had an impact on their lives. You overhear the entire conversation. What do they say?

reflect & journal

- In class, on the job, and at home, do you feel like you can fully be your authentic self? Are you living, studying, or working in a place where you find yourself coding your language or changing your actions to fit certain expectations? What keeps you from being authentic at times? Think about those expectations and their source. Now consider ways you can take steps to either share yourself more fully in these spaces or find spaces that are more supportive of your true self.

- Write a reflection on why you chose to become a nurse. Was it even a choice for you? We're guessing you've probably been asked this question a few times in nursing school, so this time, when you reflect on the "why" about your career choice, write about it in a way that gives you a sense of strength. What did you experience in your life that made you move in the direction of nursing? How did that experience make you better, stronger, and more knowledgeable about the world you live in? As you write, hang onto this journal entry and go back to it when times are tough in nursing school or your career. You can "bounce back" and remember where you came from and use that as a source of strength and resilience.

18
Providing Compassionate Care and Addressing Unmet Social Needs Can Reduce Your Burnout

—Sue Hassmiller

what

Read Chapter 18.

- There are two kinds of compassionate care described in this chapter. What do we mean when we talk about "compassionate care"?

- Only 20% of patients' health outcomes are determined by the medical care they receive (University of Wisconsin Population Health Institute, 2014). List at least six nonmedical factors that affect a patient's health.

    1. _____
    2. _____
    3. _____
    4. _____
    5. _____
    6. _____

why

What are the benefits of compassionate care? Why is compassionate care such an important component of self-care?

do

Activity 18-1: Addressing Unmet Social Needs

Much has been written about *social determinants of health*, or the social factors that have a significant impact on patients' health. These include socioeconomic status, education, neighborhoods, employment, social support, and access to healthcare (Artiga & Hinton, 2018). This chapter describes some of the ways that nurses try to address these needs with food pantries as well as partnerships with social service agencies to connect patients with vital social services. How do your local hospitals identify and address these unmet social needs? How prevalent are these issues in your community? A lot of this information will be available through your local department of health and in agencies that address specific needs, such as mental health and substance use disorders and maternal health.

Activity 18-2: Find Your Voice

In the final sidebar, Elizabeth Métraux advises: "You've found your calling, now find your voice—and your people." In this activity, we ask you to inventory your talents and skills that can become your voice as you advocate for your patients. Are you a good speaker? A compelling writer? A natural leader or persuader? When have you used these talents to effect change?

Activity 18-3: Find Your People

Next, find your people. Research advocacy groups at your institution and in your community. What issue are you especially passionate about? What are the national and international organizations that work to address this issue? Finally, learn about the advocacy work done by professional nursing and healthcare groups, such as the American Nurses Association or Partners in Health. Is there an organization that you would like to become a part of?

reflect & journal

The chapter author shares her personal story of when her husband was in a fatal accident. What behaviors did his nurses, Abby and Kathy, exhibit that made such an impact on her? What impact did Abby and Kathy's compassionate care have on their own well-being?

Métraux says it is "impossible to separate the well-being of providers from the pain endured by patients." How does it feel to know that your own well-being is woven into the well-being of those around you, especially those who may be suffering deeply? What implications does this have for you?

references

Artiga, S., & Hinton, E. (2018, May). *Beyond health care: The role of social determinants in promoting health and health equity* (Issue Brief). Henry J. Kaiser Family Foundation. https://www.kff.org/disparities-policy/issue-brief/beyond-health-care-the-role-of-social-determinants-in-promoting-health-and-health-equity/

University of Wisconsin Population Health Institute. (2014). *2014 rankings key findings report*. Robert Wood Johnson Foundation. https://www.countyhealthrankings.org/sites/default/files/2014%20County%20Health%20Rankings%20Key%20Findings.pdf

19
Showing Up With Grit and Grace: How to Lead Under Pressure as a Nurse Clinician and Leader

—Lili Powell

what

Read Chapter 19.

- How would you define *grit*? (You may also want to refer to Chapter 2.) How does Manny exhibit grit in this chapter? Provide two examples of grit that you have practiced or witnessed as a nursing student.

    1. _____
    2. _____

- How would you define *grace*? How does Manny exhibit grace? List two examples of grace that you have practiced or witnessed as a nursing student.

    1. _____
    2. _____

- What does the author mean by the term *leading mindfully*?

why

Why are grit and grace such important foundations for effective leaders? Please keep in mind that everyone is a leader, not just those at the top of the organizational charts.

do

Activity 19-1: Resilience Map

Do the same exercise that Manny did, mapping his resilience on a typical day. As you recall, he woke up tired and sluggish, went through stages of hyperarousal during work, crashed and felt irritated and exhausted toward the end of his shift, and came home with no energy left at all. Map your resilience using the example in Figure 19.4. Narrate your map. What do you notice? Are there small changes you can try with the goal of maximizing your time spent in the resilient zone?

Activity 19-2: Wrappers on the Cart

We love that Manny's story epitomizes what so many authors have shared in the textbook, including both the art of reframing and the power of perspective. Manny discovered that he had the capacity to *choose* how he perceived those wrappers on the carts each morning. The circumstance—wrappers on the carts—was always the same, but Manny's thoughts about them changed. Initially he was annoyed and irritated by them. They made him feel unappreciated and put upon. When he changed his thoughts to see the wrappers as reminders that his colleagues, too, were busy and overworked, his thoughts about the wrappers—and his colleagues—changed. He felt compassion toward his coworkers, and one result of this change was Manny's own well-being.

Do you have a pet peeve? What regularly annoys you? Reframe your personal "wrappers on the cart" and see what happens. You have the power to choose.

Activity 19-3: Arrive-Breathe-Connect

Follow the instructions for the Arrive-Breathe-Connect exercise in Chapter 19. For the next week, practice this exercise at least once a day. Which is easier for you to connect to: grit or grace?

reflect & journal

The chapter author writes that "while you perform, you are also leading, because others are consciously and unconsciously picking up on your cues. Whether or not you and others are aware of it, how you show up in the moment leads others through the power of *your* example." We don't always realize how much power we have in any given situation. We have the ability to turn everything around simply by our presence, demeanor, and grace. In the coming week, pay attention to your own power to influence those around you, hopefully in a positive way!

20
Coaching Yourself When Things Are Hard

—McKenzie Harper

what

Read Chapter 20.

- Summarize Adler's four themes of the stories we tell ourselves.

    1. _____
    2. _____
    3. _____
    4. _____

- What is the purpose of a "tiny narrative"?

- List at least two other self-coaching strategies you can use during challenging times.

    1. _____
    2. _____

why

The author embraces the phrase "Love Who You Are" in her roles as a teacher and writer. Why might this be the perfect conclusion to your self-care journey using this textbook? (We hope you will continue your journey for years to come!)

do

Activity 20-1: Write a Tiny Narrative

Be sure to try the tiny narrative exercise that the author shares in this chapter. As a reminder, here are the steps she recommends:

1. Focus on a single small moment—let's try a moment that felt difficult—and think about how it unfolded. Why did this moment matter in your life? Perhaps you sent an email to the wrong person, showed up at a party on the wrong day, or goofed up on a presentation in front of your class. Maybe you scored an "own goal" during a soccer game, but someone comforted you and that person became a good friend. The list of story possibilities is endless!

2. Try writing this story as if you were telling it to a reader with whom you can be completely yourself. Ask yourself how this moment has greater meaning or could offer a message to others. After you write one draft, try editing to limit yourself to about 100 words.

3. Now check in with yourself. Did you first frame your moment as a contamination story or a redemption story? If the former, can you (or did you) reframe it?

4. Uncomfortable with writing? Give it a try! Practice that idea of finding the positive thread, even if it feels hard to grasp.

Activity 20-2: Commit to One Practice for One Week. Start Small.

Try one or more of these strategies. Start small—maybe with the sticky notes and by developing your delight radar. Do *one thing* today. Commit to it for a week.

Meditation

Try a loving-kindness meditation. Here are a few meditation resources:

- Mindful Website: https://www.mindful.org/this-loving-kindness-meditation-is-a-radical-act-of-love
- *Wherever You Go, There You Are,* by Jon Kabat-Zinn
- Tara Brach (https://www.tarabrach.com) is a meditation teacher, psychologist, and author. You can find her guided meditations anywhere that you listen to podcasts.
- Greater Good Science Center: https://ggsc.berkeley.edu

Journaling

Keep a journal. Document your thoughts and emotions when stress arises. This not only helps you identify recurring negative patterns but also provides a tangible outlet for expressing and processing your feelings. You can do this as a note on your phone, too!

Sticky Notes (aka Positive Affirmations)

Develop a repertoire of positive phrases to counteract negative thoughts. When you catch yourself engaging in self-criticism, repeat affirmations like "You are capable," "You got this!" or "You are resilient." Even "You are beautiful" or "You are enough, just as you are." Over time, these affirmations can become powerful tools in changing your self-talk. One strategy is to post these affirmations around your home; who doesn't want to look in the bathroom mirror and see a sticky note that says, "You got this!" each morning. In fact, this would be a great thing to hop up and do right now. If you are living with roommates, they'll appreciate these notes too; your positive affirmations will have a ripple effect. If you'd like to be more private about this project, place your notes in places like your sock drawer, a book you are reading, or on your computer screen.

Go Looking for Joy: Turn on Your Delight Radar

Spend time every day noticing things that bring you joy. These can be tiny things! For example, the way your dog snores while you are working, the way the rain sounds on your roof, a delicious bite of food, or the way a colleague smiles when you walk by.

reflect & journal

The author's message to you—"Love Who You Are"—might be easy to dismiss, but you shouldn't. Find 20 minutes in a quiet place, and write all the reasons you love who you are. Are you compassionate, hardworking, or easygoing? What are the qualities that others love and admire about you? Try to stay focused on these gifts that you bring and don't wander off to areas where you think you need improvement. How does it feel to see these qualities written on the page?

Close your eyes and imagine a difficulty that you are having right now. You'll need a mental image for that difficulty (e.g., a dark cloud). Now imagine that you are at home, and you hear a knock at the door. You open the door, and staring you in the face is your difficulty. While your first instinct is to slam the door and lock it, open the door wide and invite that difficulty in. Sit with it on your couch, and ask what you can do to make it feel better. What opportunities for growth and learning exist for you?

www.ingramcontent.com/pod-product-compliance
Lightning Source LLC
Chambersburg PA
CBHW060234240426
43671CB00016B/2938